SOPHIE RANDAL

THE HIDDEN CAUSE OF ACNE

The Essential Guide on the Cause of Acne and How to
Cure it Permanently, Discover the Cause and Treatments
Available to Get Rid of Acne Permanently

Descrierea CIP a Bibliotecii Naţionale a României
SOPHIE RANDAL
    THE HIDDEN CAUSE OF ACNE. The Essential Guide on the Cause of Acne and How to Cure it Permanently, Discover the Cause and Treatments Available to Get Rid of Acne Permanently / Sophie Randal – Bucharest: Editura My Ebook, 2021
    ISBN

SOPHIE RANDAL

THE HIDDEN CAUSE OF ACNE

**The Essential Guide on the Cause of Acne and How to
Cure it Permanently, Discover the Cause and Treatments
Available to Get Rid of Acne Permanently**

My Ebook Publishing House
Bucharest, 2021

TABLE OF CONTENTS

INTRODUCTION

Acne is a common problem that is dealt with people of ages and genders. Most acne problems are typically associated with teenagers, but they are not the only people affected. In fact, even a small baby can be prone to acne breakouts.

Women and men both suffer from acne and a cure or better treatment is always being sought.

Twenty-five percent of men and fifty percent of women suffer from some form of acne whether it is blackheads and whiteheads, pimples or cysts. The severity of acne is often the cause of many psychological issues such as depression and a negative self-image. Acne is something that is hard to deal with no matter how old you are and it is very possible to suffer from acne into your forties.

The good news is that there is a lot of information on acne and ways to treat it. Each person may have different treatment requirements and sometimes you just have to try a few different products before you find the one that works for your body. Treatment can be very effective and this eBook is your guide to what acne is and how you can deal with it.

There are also a variety of homeopathic treatments and different diets that you can use to help control your acne once you find a treatment that works. Acne does not have to destroy your self-image. It is something that everyone faces at least once in their life and it is important for you to realize that there are steps you can take to improve your acne condition.

CHAPTER 1

WHAT IS ACNE?

Acne is a common skin condition that tends to appear during the teenage years. Acne usually appears on the face, but it can show up in other places as well. It is not limited to one particular area on your body. Most people will experience acne at some point in their life and it can affect you as an adult as well. Acne appears in every race and affects males and females almost equally, although women tend to suffer more frequently.

Acne Vulgaris is the proper name for acne. This condition is typically characterized by lesions that break out on the skin. The lesions can be whiteheads, blackheads or cysts which form because of clogged pores. This is commonly seen during puberty because this is when the body begins to produce an abundance of oil and a substance referred to as sebum. Sebum is required to keep the skin soft and lubricated. During puberty, however, it is produced more than needed. This excess causes the skin to feel oily and clogged pores.

Another change occurs during puberty is that the body begins to produce an excess amount of follicle cells. These dying cells will quickly build up and combine with the excess sebum that is being produced. This combination produces whiteheads. The area and mixture is a prime breeding ground for bacteria, which results in redness and swelling in the area. This inflammation is known as a pimple. Blackheads and whiteheads are non-inflamed areas, although they can be seen if grouped together closely.

Acne is extremely common condition that affects about 85% of people, especially between the ages of 12 and 24. About a quarter of this group will experience acne not only on their face, but on their back as well their neck. About 40% of people will seek medical attention for severe acne.

The main area for acne breakouts on the face is referred to as the "T-Zone." This zone includes the forehead, nose and chin. Acne may appear on the cheeks and other parts of the face, but these areas tend to be much oilier than other areas. The next most common areas are the back, the neck, the chest and then the shoulders.

What's Inside a Pimple?

A pimple is, by definition, a red, raised bump that is clogged with oil and dead skin and is infected with bacteria. The pimple bursts beneath the skin and sends the bacteria into the surrounding tissue. It is then called a papule. If this spreads deeper into the skin it is called a papule. If it goes even deeper it is then called a pustule. A pustule is not usually as red as other pimples, but it may have a white center and be painful. If it goes deeper than a pustule, then it is called a cyst. A cyst can be very serious needs to be treated by a trained professional.

Propionibacterium acne is found on the skin. This type of acne usually increases during puberty, as it uses sebum as a nutrient. Some people may have even more bacteria on their skin. When this occurs it collects in the pore of the hair follicle and becomes clogged with dead cells, a comedone is formed. A comedone is the medical term for blackheads and whiteheads. After the whitehead is formed, the body sends white blood cells to the follicle. The white blood cells begin to fight the bacteria and try to destroy it. This causes inflammation in the area.

A normal follicle has sebum that is produced by your sebaceous glands. The sebum fills the hair follicle and spreads over your skin; this is what causes skin to appear oily. When the cells slough off after dying, they may become lodged in the hair follicle with the sebum. If the oil breaks through to the surface, then you will see a whitehead. If the oxygen oxidizes the oil, then the comedone changes from white to black and you see a blackhead.

You shouldn't pick at or pop pimples, but sometimes they are painful and you have to relieve the pressure. There is a sanitary way to do this that we will share with you later. In the meantime you are wondering what comes out of the pimple when you pop it – right? What you see is a whitish-yellow fluid. The fluid contains white blood cells, old tissue that has become liquefied and other cellular debris. This pus is often the site of infection where a foreign body has entered the body. This stuff is perfectly natural for it to be found in a pimple. The pus is the result of your body trying to fight off the bacteria.

Hormones Causing Acne

Testosterone often causes acne to appear in athletes who use performance- enhancing drugs. Acne fulminansis is caused by testosterone and can have various affects on the body that would not normally be contributed to acne. Symptoms may include:

- Severe scarring
- Painful joints
- Rising and falling fever
- Decreased appetite
- Weight loss
- Quick onset of acne

Scarring is often found with people who have suffered from acne fulminansis. This comes from collagen that is formed to heal the cells that have been injured by acne. This often results in excessive scarring.

Testosterone comes from cholesterol and is produced in the testes of the man. Women produce small amounts of testosterone in ovaries. Testosterone flows through the body and then binds to the androgen receptors. Both men and women have androgen receptors but the two sexes respond to them differently. Testosterone is not only the cause of acne in athletes and it doesn't have to be performance-enhancing. Testosterone is often the cause of formation of acne at puberty. It can also affect women later in life as well. At puberty, the testosterone levels rise and causes the body to increase its sebum production and increases the oiliness of skin and hair, causing outbreaks.

Migrating Acne

Body acne is another condition that is suffered by many people and it just goes to show that acne is not restricted to the face. Body acne affects both teenagers and adults. It may appear on their back, neck and shoulders. It can also appear on the chest and buttocks. There are several factors that can cause this acne to occur including:

- Tight fitting clothing
- Perspiration
- Clothing that can't "breathe"

People who are physically active are often prone to body acne. This is especially true if they wear clothing such as spandex. Spandex traps fluids against the skin and causes it to block the hair follicles and pores.

Body acne can be similar to facial acne, but it can show up in some awkward places. Skin that is located on the body is often thicker and more susceptible to friction that is caused by clothing that fits tightly and rubs on the skin.

CHAPTER 2

TYPES OF ACNE

There are several forms of acne that can range from mild to severe. It can be found on various parts of the body. Mild acne can be self-treated, but severe cases are best treated by a dermatologist or health professional. The most common type of acne is "common acne," such as Acne Vulgaris. This type of acne includes your typical whiteheads, blackheads, pustules, papules, nodules and cysts.

Blackheads

Blackheads, or comedones, occur in pores that are partially blocked. Sebum, dead cells and bacteria will slowly drain to the surface of the poor and then the black color is caused by the skin pigment being exposed to air. These often take a long time to clear up.

Whiteheads

Whiteheads are comedones as well, but they are somewhat different than blackheads. These are caused by pores that are completely blocked and stuck under the surface of the skin.

Papules

Papules are small red bumps on your skin. These tend to be very tender and cause irritation. These may cause scarring, so try not to touch or squeeze these.

Pustules

These red bumps are what we know as pimples or zits. They appear as a red circle with a white or yellow center.

Nodules

Nodules are much larger than other forms of acne. These are hard lumps that appear beneath the surface of the skin, which can be very painful and last for a great deal of time. This type of acne is very vulnerable to scarring and it is advisable to have them treated by a dermatologist.

Cysts

These are very similar to nodules, except that they are filled with pus. These are often painful and may scar if left untreated. These should also be treated by a dermatologist.

Acne Conglobata

This is a relatively rare form of acne vulgaris. It can be disfiguring and cause severe suffering both psychologically and physically. These are often very large lesions that form on your face, chest, buttocks, back, upper arms and thighs. It is also accompanied by blackheads. This often causes damage and permanent scarring. This is often a condition that appears more in men than in women. This condition is known to persist for several years.

Acne Fulminans

This is often the sudden appearance of Acne Conglobata and is accompanied by a fever and achy joints. This is usually treated with oral steroids.

Gram-Negative Folliculitis

This condition can be caused by long-term treatment of acne with antibiotics and is a bacterial infection, which causes cysts and pustules.

Pyoderma Faciale

This is a type of acne that affects females between the ages of 20 and 40. This can cause very painful pustules, nodules and cysts. They appear on the face and leave a permanent scarring. This often occurs in women who have never experienced acne before and often clears up in about a year.

Acne Rosacea

This type of acne tends to appear in people who are over the age of 30. This is a red rash that appears on cheeks, forehead, nose and chin. There may also be pimples and other blemishes. This tends to occur more in women than in men.

When men do breakout with it, it tends to be more severe. This is much different than Acne Vulgaris and requires a different treatment.

Baby Acne

Baby acne often manifests itself as white bumps that appear on the baby's body. This is really nothing to worry about and it is very natural. Baby acne is traced back to the hormones that pass through the placenta to the baby. The condition may also develop several days or weeks after birth. When the baby receives the surge of hormones right before birth, they often develop baby acne.

This condition can be soothed with a mild soap and lukewarm water once per day. Do not use lotions or oils as it may aggravate the skin. You also want to avoid excessive cleansing and scrubbing. Baby acne is not caused by dirt or debris so scrubbing doesn't help.

Acne Dysmorphia

This is not technically a physical condition caused by acne, but it is a mental condition. This can be a very debilitating illness that may show up with someone who has a preoccupation with deformity. In this situation the person is totally preoccupied with acne. They believe that their acne is horrible and that their skin is awful, when in actuality it may not be all that bad. They are often preoccupied by checking themselves in a mirror and obsessively checking on their skin flaws.

Billions of people have acne outbreaks, but these people are unable to deal with it. In fact, this disorder has nothing to do with acne. This disorder is also related to anorexia nervosa. In anorexia, weight is a trigger; in acne dysmorphia, acne is a trigger. These people are obsessed with their skin and it is not unusual for this type of person to continuously look in the mirror and obsess about their skin.

Acne dysmorphia has been successfully treated with serotonin reuptake inhibitors as well as hypnosis. Cognitive Behavioral Therapy is a psychological treatment for depression related disorders. Group therapy sessions with people who suffer from similar problems have allowed people to relieve themselves from the obsession that they suffer from. People with this condition have also been treated with antidepressants and other medications.

Scalp Folliculitis

Scalp folliculitis is when the pores on your scalp become clogged. This condition has a variety of names, but it is simply scalp acne. Scalp acne can affect anybody of any age. This type of acne is limited to just the scalp either. In fact, it can show up anywhere hair follicles are located including:

- Armpits
- Arms
- Leg
- Face

These are small pustules that are of a whitish-yellow color. Hair will often grow straight through these pustules. When you pick at them, they may ooze with sebum and bloodstained pus. The hair may also grow right next to the area, but the pustule is still in the hair follicle. This condition tends to be somewhat itchy and people find it hard not to touch them. The pustules can be located anywhere on the scalp, but often only affects a small area.

This problem is formed the same way that acne is formed. This acne involves a bacterium that becomes trapped in the hair follicle. *P. acnes* is often the culprit in this problem. Staphylococcus bacterium is also known to cause this condition.

Staphylococcus bacterium is known to cause other problems such as eye and nose infections.

Some people may develop scalp folliculitis when they sit in hot tubs or other warm and moist locations that are not chlorinated. The temperature softens the scalp and allows the hair follicles to be more susceptible to bacteria and infection. Ingrown hairs also cause it, as they are the perfect breeding grown for this bacterium. Other causes include:

- Diabetes
- Excessive sweating
- Tight clothing

- Unsanitary conditions
- Exposure to both heat and humidity
- Dermatitis
- Eczema
- Flu and colds

Scalp folliculitis is contagious and can be passed from one person to another. People need to be certain to use clean towels. Don't share items such as:

- Towels
- Brushes
- Combs
- Hair Accessories
- Pillow cases

If scalp folliculitis is a persistent problem, be sure to visit a doctor. They will help you to determine if the infection is caused by a bacteria or fungus, which is another factor that can cause this condition. They will help you find an appropriate treatment plan as well. Many doctors will prescribe an over the counter cream that is applied to the area daily. These treatments may be Bacitracin, Neomycin and Mycitracin. These are applied three to four times per day.

CHAPTER 3

ACNE TREATMENTS

There are a variety of different treatments available to those suffering from acne. Some treatments such as home treatments are generally good for mild cases of acne, but when it comes to severe acne you are better off seeing a doctor or dermatologist.

Home Treatments

Home treatments essentially begin with washing your face. However, this simple task you have probably done most of your life may actually be causing you more problems than preventing them. Washing your face with a specially formulated soap can help to prevent acne. If you wash your face several times per day, then you may actually be washing away skin oils that are essential to your skin. This causes the sebaceous glands to produce more oil and cause problems.

Scrubbing on your face can actually cause you to create acne problems by scrubbing way the essential oils and damaging hair follicles.

Water is a simple home treatment as well. Water carries nutrients throughout your body and can be very effective in helping you to clear up acne flare-ups. Your bowels and kidneys store the toxins from everything that you eat and breathe. These toxins can cause acne flare-ups as well. By drinking six to eight glass of water per day, you are able to flush out toxins from your bowels and kidneys.

Herbs are also recommended to acne sufferers. Black currant seed oil and evening primrose oil are very popular with acne sufferers. It is suggested that you take three 500mg capsules per day.

Vitamins

Most people are deficient in essential vitamins and minerals that your body needs to work properly. Your skin needs the proper nutrition to work and to prevent skin conditions such as acne. Vitamins and minerals are essential and can help to flush out free radicals and toxins in your body. Other vitamins have antibacterial effects that aid the immune system in fighting off infection and bacteria.

Vitamin A will help to strengthen and protect your skin. It helps to reduce the production of sebum and then aids in the repair of tissues. It can also be a powerful antioxidant. These are important and required to help you rid your body of toxins. A lack of vitamin A can actually cause acne.

The Complex B vitamins are also essential in preserving healthy skin. They can aid in reducing stress, as it is believed to be a common source of acne problems. The B vitamins should be taken together. They include Thiamine, Riboflavin, Niacinamide, Pantothenic Acid (B5) and Pyriodixine (B6). These vitamins play a large role in digestion, stress reduction, and improving circulation.

Vitamin C has been referred to as the "super vitamin." It aids in approximately 300 metabolic functions in your body. It is also essential in tissue growth, tissue repair, and flushes toxins from your system. It can also improve immunity and fight against infection. Persons with diabetes should check with their doctors before taking vitamin C.

Chromium is often used for weight loss, but it can also help fight acne. It should be taken in an added form, as it is difficult to absorb chromium from foods. A large amount of chromium is lost in the digestion of sugar.

Zinc aids in regulating the activity of oil glands. It promotes healing in tissues and prevents scarring. Zinc also helps to strengthen the immune system and the healing of wounds. In addition, it is a powerful antioxidant that prevents the formation of free radicals and toxins.

A multivitamin with chromium will often supply your body with the nutrients it needs to fight acne. It is recommended that you take a multivitamin twice per day. It is almost impossible for the body to get all of the nutrients it needs from a multivitamin when it is only taken once a day.

Blue Light Therapy

This is an alternative therapy that is aimed for those who suffer from acne but have had little success in treating it. This therapy focuses on killing off the bacteria that causes acne formation. This bacterium is called propionibacterium acnes or *P. acnes*. *P. acnes* causes small molecules to produce bacteria that causes most types of acne. These molecules are known as porphyrins and blue light therapy works to zero in on the porphyrins. When these molecules are exposed to blue light, they produce free radicals that destroy the bacteria.

This treatment is becoming very popular because it is both non-invasive and drug free. Many medications contain chemicals that cause damage to the skin. This therapy does not cause this and it is FDA approved and safe for the skin. Blue light therapy is administered in increments. A patient is put on a schedule for several short 15-minute sessions over a period of about 4 weeks.

Light and Heat Energy Therapy

This is another form of light energy that has been used to treat acne. It uses both light and heat to eradicate the cause of acne. It also destroys the acne causing bacteria and reduces the production of sebum. This helps to shrink the sebaceous glands. Improvements are often seen as early as 30 days and sessions are as short as 10 minutes. This therapy has also been approved by the FDA, but it is used to treat mild to moderate acne.

Laser Light Therapy

Laser light therapy is another effective way of preventing scarring with chronic acne cases. It has also been used in healing breakouts as well. After a few treatments with a nonabrasive laser surgery, the scars that remain from bad acne breakouts can be treated. This is due to the collage growth that is promoted under the scars. Treatments range from five to twenty minutes and there is usually only slight discomfort. There is marked improvement in skin after only a few treatments. There are a few side effects such as mild redness and swelling for a short amount of time, but it does not interfere with the patient's life.

Over the Counter (OTC) Treatments

Just about everyone purchases an over the counter treatment and many people have varying success. If acne is mild and infrequent then these products will usually work. Those people with sever problems usually do not find much help from these products.

When choosing an over the counter treatment you will need to look at the active ingredient. Not all products will work in the same manner because of their ingredients. One of the most common active ingredients is Benzoyl peroxide.

This treatment has been deemed the "wonder drug" in the acne treatment industry. This product aids in reducing the *P. acnes* bacteria and reduces the number of dead skin cells. This product helps lessen the effects of the two main causes of

28

comedones and pimples. This product has been used for several years. When it is over used, it will often dry out the skin.

Resorcinol is another ingredient that works best on small acne blemishes. It is often combined with sulfur. Sulfur itself has often been found to be an effective acne treatment for some people, it does not seem to be known why it helps to clear up acne.

Salicylic acid is found in many products and works on blemishes that are free of inflammation. It aids in unclogging pores and reduces the number of blemishes that appear. It is able to do this by minimizing dead skin cells. It does not seem to have an effect on the production of sebum or *P. acnes* bacteria. This product does cause some irritation in some people.

Remember to keep your skin type in mind. If you have sensitive skin, then you will want to take it easy with strong acne medication. This medication can easily make your problems worse rather than fix them. If your acne seems too hard to control yourself, then you need to see a doctor.

Accutane

Accutane (Isotretinoin) is one of the most famous and most controversial acne treatments on the market. This drug is often considered to be the "last resort" for people who suffer from acne and have tried everything else. The drug was first introduced in 1982 by the Hoffman-LaRoche pharmaceutical company. This product has been frequently prescribed to people who suffer from acute acne and severe nodular acne. These people have usually tried several topical treatments that have not been successful for them.

Accutane is actually a vitamin A analog. It ranges in dosage from 10mg to 40mg. The drug is very potent and after four or five months of regular use, the person will see a noticeable difference in their acne. Accutane shuts down the oil production of your skin. It forces sebaceous glands to mature. This process begins by testosterone forcing the sebaceous gland to produce different types of oils that line the hair follicle. When the oil production is stabilized, it is no longer able to clog pores. It also prevents too much keratin to be produce and clog the pores. It can take up to two months for you to see a difference. It is recommended that people take Accutane with fatty foods, such as milk. This allows the drug to be easily absorbed.

Accutane does have a number of drawbacks. Users often experience a worsening of symptoms before they see improvement. They may also experience dry skin, lips and eyes. It has also been linked to several birth defects and should not be taken by women who are pregnant. Women may also need to use two types of contraception when on Accutane. It may also cause depression and digestive problems.

Accutane has been pretty successful. About 35-38% of patients will experience complete remission after one course. People with severe, stubborn acne may need more than one course. After one course, 70% of people have experienced remission of symptoms. One course of treatment is usually about four to six months.

Birth Control

Many adult women suffer from acne. In response to this, many women have found that low dose birth control is able to help clear up their skin as well. One type of birth control pill that has been proven to be effective is Ortho Tri-Cyclen. It is able to reduce androgens and regulate female hormones so that the changes in hormones do not cause acne outbreaks. Some women are more prone to these hormonal changes and are sensitive to hormones and high levels of testosterone. A woman's oil glands may respond to these changes in hormones and cause outbreaks. The hormone balancing birth control plan has been proven in many studies. Women need to consider the side effects that are associated with birth control pills before taking on this type of plan.

Cryotherapy

Cryotherapy is available through dermatologists. This option includes the use of liquid nitrogen or solid carbon dioxide to be applied to an area of skin. These substances freeze the skin. Lightly freezing the skin causes it to peel. Moderate freezing will cause it to blister and hard freezing will cause it to scab over. This procedure has also been used to remove scars and cancerous growths. These substances are sprayed on or swabbed. This is one of the most inexpensive ways to remove surface skin lesions. The skin is lightly frozen so that the top layer is shed and the accompanying comedones are removed as well. This treatment has also been used to cause pimples to heal more quickly and to reduce scarring.

These treatments are usually performed once a week. Side effects may include stinging and redness. The area may also be tender and painful afterwards.

Steroid creams are often prescribed for use after treatment. This treatment has been available since the 60s and has been very effective.

Choosing a Dermatologist

When you suffer from severe acne or acne that is very painful, you will need to consider going to a dermatologist. Your self-esteem will probably thank you for this, and you will need to consider several concepts to ensure that you are choosing the best doctor for your needs.

Most people feel apprehensive when they visit a dermatologist for the first time. They feel very odd about having somebody go and pick around at your face.

You will also be showing off things that you spend a lot of time trying to hide as well. When you begin "shopping around" for a dermatologist, you will want to make a list of what you are looking for and what your concerns are. You want to find someone who is concerned with your needs and your mental stability, versus someone who is mostly concerned with your acne instead of you. Consider these few questions:

- What do you like about your primary physician?
- Are you concerned about someone who is sensitive to your concerns?
- Do you want someone with a good bedside manner?

- Are you worried that appointments won't accommodate your hectic schedule?

Whatever your needs are, a good dermatologist will answer your questions and will do their best to be sensitive to your needs. They will also be able to provide you with a variety of treatment options. If you have any questions about available treatments they should be able to answer those questions as well. Be open and honest with your dermatologist and they will do the same for you. They want you to be prepared for the treatment and they want to offer all of the information you can. If you are nervous, tell your doctor and they will do their best to help you out.

A well-trained dermatologist will be a medical doctor that is board certified and trained in dermatology. The dermatologist should also be a member of the American Academy of Dermatology. You will also need to find a dermatologist with experience in dealing with acne and the severity that you may have. An experienced dermatologist is able to give you a more accurate diagnosis and will provide you with an appropriate treatment.

Scar Removal and Treatment

Acne scars are the result of tissue damage cause by acne that was left untreated or treated improperly. When the tissue is damaged, the body reacts by initiating the repair process and causes collagen to build up in the damaged area. This excess collagen causes a fibrous mass that ends up becoming a smooth, but firm scar. The scars may also result when the tissue has been lost and is the most common type of scar. There are several different categories of scars including:

- "Ice-pick" scar
- Depressed scars
- Soft scars
- Atrophic macules

Scars are treated through a variety of different options. One effective method is to inject collagen into the site of the scar. This is a process that has to be repeated about every three to six months. The collagen will cause the skin to puff and makes the scar less noticeable.

Another process that is similar involves using a person's own body fat. This is called an autologus fat transfer. The fat is taken from another part of the body and then injected into the acne scar. It causes the scar to fill out. This process will also need to be repeated because the fat is reabsorbed.

Dermabrasion is another common method for treating scarring. This is done under local anesthesia. During this process, a thin layer of skin is removed using a fraise or brush at high speed. This removes the surface layer and can actually remove some shallow scarring. This can lessen the depth of the scarring.

Microdemabrasion removes the skin surface using crystals of aluminum oxide that is passed through a vacuum.

CHAPTER 4

PREVENTING ACNE & ACNE MYTHS BUSTED

It was once believed that acne was caused by poor hygiene. This fact has long been overthrown, as it has been discovered that it can actually cause acne to become worse. Prevention does include proper hygiene, but here is the rest of the story that many people don't know.

Does Your Diet Affect Acne?

It has long been believed that foods that are fried, chocolate or soda cause acne. Well, this great debate is over because it has been shown that these items have no scientific root linking them to acne.

There is no scientific evidence that shows that foods such as pizza, French fries or soda cause acne. Acne is caused by a biomechanism that causes your sebaceous glands to produce too much oil. These oils are much different than those that are used in cooking food. This myth has been around for so long because people simply believe that it is true. They cease eating foods and their skin clears up, but this can be due to a variety of other physical effects. Some people have noticed these changes and a doctor will simply tell you that if you think that is the cause then stop eating those foods. They are not going to tell you that chocolate and Dr Pepper cause acne.

It is, however, very important that you do eat healthy. There are numerous nutrition related issues that may be caused when you don't eat a healthy diet. What you eat will not directly affect your skin, but it can cause a variety of other health problems that are much more serious than acne, such as heart disease. A balanced diet will also leave you feeling better all around. You will have more energy, slow down the effects of aging and make a healthier environment for your skin.

Acne is Not Caused by Poor Hygiene

This myth seems to make sense, but it really is not true. Acne is caused by an overproduction of sebum. This is natural oil that is essential to your skin to keep it waterproof and hydrated. A lack of cleanliness does not cause acne. In fact, the products that cause acne are located deep inside tissues that you can't clean. Over cleaning and scrubbing your skin too much or using harsh chemicals on your skin can cause you to irritate your skin, thus increasing your chances of acne.

Proper skin care is important at all times throughout your life. If you have acne, then you want to take special care to keep your skin clean and healthy. This means that you need to protect it from too much sun and harsh cosmetics.

To clean your skin you will want to use a gentle soap or specialized skin cleaner. Wash your face with this product twice per day. Don't scrub and aggravate the acne but clean it with a nice, soft cloth. Apply cleanser to all areas around the hairline and the neck. Rinse clean with water and pat dry your face. If you have very oily skin, then you may need to use an astringent. Use it only in the oily parts of your skin because dry skin will increase its oil production and make your acne worse. Hair care is also important and you will want to shampoo at least two or three times per week. If you have oily hair, then you will want to shampoo daily. This can help prevent scalp acne as well. Try to keep the shampoo off of your face as much as possible.

Tanning was once considered an acne treatment, but it really only dries out your skin and temporarily hides your acne. As your skin becomes accustomed to the sun, the acne will adjust and flare again. You are also risking skin damage and increasing your chances of skin cancer. Many acne medications are also prone to causing skin to be more sensitive to sunlight. This means you will need to be diligent about using sunscreen when outdoors.

The best thing you can do for your skin is not wear any make-up at all, but since we know this is not happening for many women, you will want to make your make-up selections carefully. Look for make-up that is "noncomedogenic" and avoid make-up that has an oil base. Be sure to read labels carefully when shopping. Be aware that even if it says "noncomedogenic," it may still cause acne in some people. Be sure to wash away all make-up every evening before you go to bed. This allows your skin to breathe and provides your acne with air. You can also look for make-up that contains products that will aid in killing bacteria that contributes to acne. In fact, this make-up can be useful in prevention as well. If you apply moderate amounts of make-up, you may be doing your skin some good. There are also several types of make-up that contain sunscreen to help prevent your face from damaging sunrays.

Avoid products that cause your skin to become dry. Avoid products that contain alcohol, as it will dry out your skin and defeat the purpose. It may kill the bacteria, but it will cause your body to produce more oil. You also want to ensure that your aftershave and perfume is as alcohol free as possible. Use products that contain a moisturizing product. Use moisturizers that are oil-free, you will also want to use oil-free foundation.

Antibacterial products will help kill the bacteria that causes acne. There are several antibacterial cleansers available that will aid in killing the bacteria. Look for products that contain Benzoyl peroxide. Be aware, however, that these can cause your skin to dry out if they are overused.

If you have long hair, you will want to sleep with your hair up and on a pillowcase that nobody else has used. This will keep the oil from your hair from causing an increased amount of oil on your face.

Shaving with acne can be uncomfortable. If you do need to use a regular razorblade to shave, then be careful around blemishes. Be sure to use plenty of water and shaving cream. Electric razors are often good because they do not scrape the skin, but cut the hairs.

Sometimes acne is caused by simply touching your skin too much. If you sit with your chin in your hand all day, don't be surprised when your chin breaks out. If you constantly swipe hair off of your forehead, don't be surprised when your forehead breaks out. By touching your face you are introducing dirt and oil to these sensitive areas.

If you have a blackhead problem on your forehead, nose or chin, there are several strips available to help you remove this debris. You simply get your skin wet, apply the strip and allow it to dry. After the strip has dried, you simply peel it off of your skin. This is an interesting sensation, but you can almost feel all of that material coming out of your pores. These are safe and very effective. They may not get them all, but if you look at the strip you will see little black spikes all over the sticky side of the strips.

Medications that Aggravate or Create Acne

There are several medications that can do you more harm than good. When this comes to your acne, you want to avoid any that may make your situation worse. Many of these medications will aggravate your already existing acne or may cause you to breakout.

Any illness may aggravate your acne or cause you to breakout. In this sort of situation, it is difficult to determine what the cause of the breakout is. Is it the illness? Medication?

Despite this fact, you want to be certain that you don't stop taking a medication that is essential for your health simply because it is causing your acne to be worse. Instead, consult your doctor to prescribe you a different medication that may be easier on your acne. It is more important that you sustain your health so that you can live even if you don't look the best you have ever looked. Acne may be painful to look at, but it is not life threatening.

Other medications that are known to cause acne include:

- **Anticonvulsants:** Certain anticonvulsants are prescribed for people who suffer from epilepsy and seizures. They may also be prescribed to people who suffer from bi-polar disorder and depression. These medications often list acne as a side effect. Lithium is another medication that is popular for these conditions and can also cause acne

- **Corticosteroids**: These are often used to treat asthma and other chronic lung disease. These medications are similar to cortisol and can stimulate the body to produce sebum, which can cause an increase in acne.

- **Sobriety Medications:** Antabuse is often prescribed to help alcoholics stop drinking. I can also cause acne in recovering alcoholics.

- **Immunosuppressants:** These types of drugs suppress the immune system. These may be required for people who have recently received an organ transplant. It can also suppress your ability to fight the bacteria that causes breakouts.

- **Thyroid Preparations:** Many thyroid medications are known to trigger acne. Large amounts of iodine may also cause breakouts.

- **Systemic Steroids:** Systemic steroids are synthetic versions of natural steroid. These may cause breakout of acne while curing another skin condition.

- **Anabolic Steroids:** These are steroids that can cause severe cases of acne in some users.

- **Cosmetic and Acne:** Acne that is caused by cosmetics is called "acne cosmetica." This acne is triggered by cosmetic products rather than the natural causes that typically cause acne. If you think that you are experiencing a breakout because of a product then you will want to discontinue using it.

- **Birth Control & Acne:** There are several oral contraceptives that may control acne but there are also several others that may cause it as well. These tend to have a low estrogen content and a progestins that increases androgens in the body. Only women are affected, obviously as it is oral contraceptive, but they tend to only be women who have a tendency towards androgenicity. Some of the pills that you may want to steer away from include:

- Loestrin 1.5/30
- Loestrin 1.5/20 Fe
- Estrostep Fe
- Levlen
- Alesse
- Ovral
- Norlestrin 1/50

Stress Does Not Make Acne Worse

Many people believe that acne is related to stress. This is simply not true because there are many stressed out individuals who are not breaking out with acne. Everybody has stress and it is a part of life. It is also a part of adolescence. Acne may cause you to become more stressed out because it is there, but it does not directly cause stress.

CONCLUSION

Acne is a part of life, but it is something that should be taken seriously. This condition can have a devastating effect on teenagers and this certainly needs to be considered if you have a teenager suffering from acne.

Parents have usually experienced the mental distress that acne can cause, so you want to be compassionate. As adults, you know that the acne will pass, but when you are in high school it can be hard to deal with. We know that people don't walk around staring down your blemishes and making fun of you, but it's still a hard part of life.

There are several new medications and treatments that you can take advantage of whether you are a teenager or an adult. There are several common conditions that can be brought under control rather quickly with this new technology.

Always consult a dermatologist if the acne is severe. You will not want this condition to go untreated, as it can prevent scarring. Scars can be a reminder of your adolescent years, which most teenagers will not want to remember. A dermatologist will be able to provide you with numerous treatment options.

Remind teenagers and yourself that acne is treatable and you are not alone in your suffering. Many people suffer from acne and, in fact, about 85% of adolescents suffer from acne. If you are unable to be successful with over the counter medications, look for professional treatment to aid you in your fight against acne.

Printed by Libri Plureos GmbH in Hamburg,
Germany